IVF FAQS ANSWERED

FOR YOUR IVF JOURNEY

DR. VINOD KUMAR N

Dedicated to all my patients, who have been very kind to me throughout my journey as an IVF specialist and also have given me these frequently asked questions which helped me complete this book without which it would not have been an easy task.

Contents

Foreword

I wrote this book to address most of the questions,
      an infertile couple ask an IVF specialist before, during and
and
      after the procedure to help ease out their anxiety.
      I hope it will help many couples who are undergoing or
      will undertake IVF journey.

Preface

IVF FAQs ANSWERED as a resource for infertility patients, will be a companion for successful treatment journey.

Written in an easy-to-read format it provides answers to the most commonly asked questions about infertility, IVF and post IVF period.

About the author, Dr Vinod Kumar N, is a MBBS graduate from Bangalore Medical College affiliated to

Rajiv Gandhi University Of Health Sciences Bangalore, is a MD(OBG) post graduate of Darbhanga Medical

College from Bihar, and has done DRME Diploma in reproductive medicine and embryology from Kiel university Germany. He has been practicing in corporate hospitals in Bangalore since 2011.

Acknowledgements

I thank everyone who supported me in writing this book.

I want to thank you and congratulate you for purchasing/downloading the book. The book contains answers for most of the frequently asked questions, and will help you in your journey towards parenthood as a companion. This book will provide you the right information which will increase your chances of achieving your dream to have a baby. If you are considering IVF, then this is the material for you. Thanks again for downloading this book, I hope you will be happy after reading this book.

Prologue

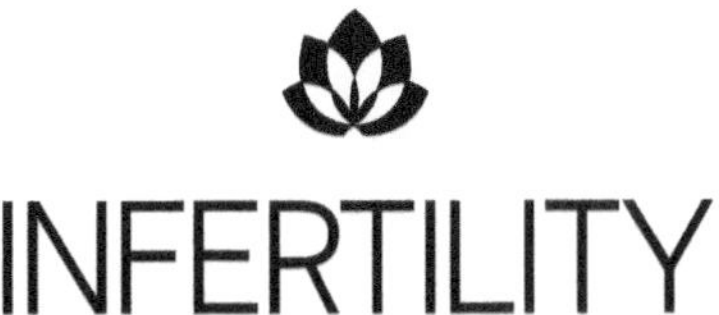

CHAPTER ONE

INFERTILITY

What is INFERTILITY ?

If you are trying regularly to get pregnant from past 12 months, without using any contraceptive methods and unable to conceive, it is called as Infertility. One in six couples in India have difficulty getting pregnant.

Being infertile does not mean that you will never have children, just that you need assistance in finding the cause of the problem and ivf specialist help with treatment to resolve it.

What causes INFERTILITY ?

Infertility can be caused by a number of factors in both women and men.

In women, the most common factors are due to problems of ovulation, blocked or damaged fallopian tubes, endometriosis, adenomiosis, uterine problems, Increasing age etc.

In men, the most common factors are low sperm count, less motile sperms, minor genetic problems that affect sperm count and quality, past infection, lifestyle factors like excessive smoking or alcohol consumption, etc, or sometimes a combination of factors in both the partners.

Unexplained infertility

In some couples we can't find an obvious cause, and this is termed "unexplained infertility".

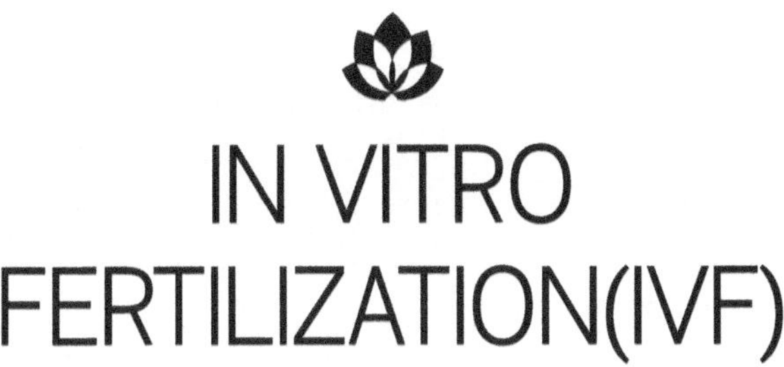

CHAPTER TWO

IN VITRO FERTILIZATION(IVF)

What are the steps of IVF ?

1. Stimulation of eggs.

Hormonal Injections are given to the woman for growth of eggs.

2. Ovum pick up (OPU).

Eggs are aspirated out of the ovary through a small needle under anaesthesia.

3. IVF/ICSI for fertilization.

What is In vitro fertilization (IVF) ?

In IVF, the sperms and the eggs are allowed to fertilize in a small petri dish to form embryos, when semen analysis is normal.

What is Intra cytoplasmic sperm injection (ICSI) ?

In ICSI, each sperm is injected into the egg with the help of a fine needle, when the semen analysis report shows problems in count, motility & morphology.

When is IVF Needed ?

It was originally developed for women with blocked or missing fallopian tubes, it can also be done for conditions such as female factor infertility, male factor infertility and unexplained infertility. An IVF specialist reviews a patient's history and guides them to the diagnostic procedures and treatment that is appropriate for the couple.

4. Blastocyst culture.

Embryos are cultured in an incubator to develop, and usually transferred 2-3 days after egg collection. Blastocyst culture involves allowing embryos to mature further upto 'Day 5' in an incubator before embryo transfer or freezing of embryos.

5. Freezing of embryos.

Storage of embryos at -196 degree Celsius, so that they are kept for longer duration.

6. Embryo transfer.

Embryos are loaded into a syringe and then transferred into the uterus under ultrasound guidance.

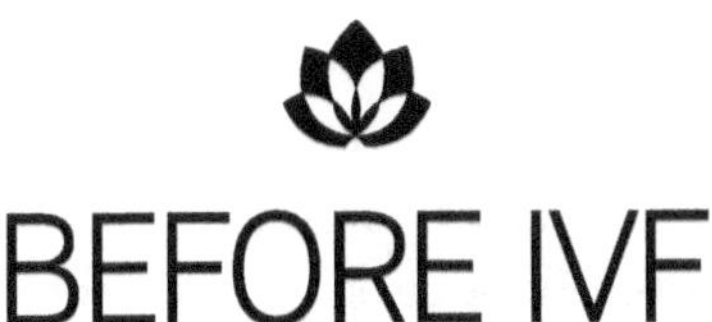

BEFORE IVF

1. How long does an IVF treatment process take ?

If everything goes as expected and planned, usually it takes between 4 and 6 weeks, from the start of your treatment till the result in fresh embryo transfer cycle. It takes a lil longer if it is a Frozen embryo transfer cycle.

2. How many days of hospitalisation is required for ?

No need of hospitalisation throughout ivf procedure.

3. How many hospital visits will be there during the treatment ?

Multiple visits are required throughout treatment process. Initially 1-2 visits for the basic tests, and then for a continious 10-12 days during stimualtion and opu phase, following which the visits reduce till embryo transfer.

4. Does my partner have to visit to the clinic ?

We will need to see both the partners at the initial consultation in order to take your past medical history and schedule baseline blood tests and other investigations required for each of them.

5. When should be the first visit to the hospital ?

First visit can be on any menstrual day, but for stimulation of eggs you will be asked to come on second day of your menstruation.

6. What constitutes day one of my cycle?

Day one of your cycle is considered your first day of menstrual bleeding, not spotting. If this occurs after 12 p.m., then the next day is considered day one.

7. Can a woman who has attained Menopause undergo IVF ?

yes a woman who has attained Menopause, also can undergo IVF with Donor eggs.

8. Till what age women can opt for IVF ?

Presently in india, Upto 45 years of women age, one can opt for IVF.

9. What are the basic tests done to start IVF ?

Basic blood test for both the couple, pelvic ultrasound for woman and semen analysis for for the husband.

For men with abnormal semen results, we may suggest other blood tests, genetic studies and testicular exploration.

10. Is laparoscopy procedure, a mandatory test before IVF ?

No laparoscopy is not a mandatory test for before IVF.

11. Is endometrial biopsy test for Tuberculosis, mandatory before IVF ?

No endometrial biopsy for tuberculosis is not mandatory before IVF but if the treating doctor suspects tuberculosis in woman then it may be advised.

12. Is HSG a mandatory test before IVF ?

No HSG is not a mandatory test before IVF but if HSG shows bilateral fallopian tube blockage then IVF is the treatment of choice.

13. Who will give me the injections ?

Usually one of the nursing staff from the hospital will give injections. But you, or a family member, can also be taught by our staff how to give the subcutaneous injections at home, if you dont wish you visit hospital.

14. Are IVF injections painful ?

Hormonal njections are a part of IVF treatment, medicines that once had to be injected into the muscle have been replaced by medicines given under the skin (subcutaneous) to minimize discomfort and stress.

After OPU, patients are given a progesterone hormone supplement in order to prepare the lining of the uterus for the embryo transfer. For most patients, progesterone may be taken in a vaginal tablet or vaginal suppository rather than an injection so that, injections may be avoided entirely during the second half of the IVF cycle.

15. What are the side effects of the medicines, I will be taking ?

IVF treatment side effects vary from patient to patient. However, reactions to medications may include skin irritation at the injection site, abdominal bloating, headaches, breast tenderness, and nausea.

16. Are there any long term side effects due to hormonal medicines during IVF ?

In general population, women who have never conceived have a slightly increased risk of ovarian cancer. Because it is thought that many of these women have used fertility medicines, it may cause ovarian cancer.

A number of studies have been conducted, have found **no association** between fertility medicines and higher risk of ovarian cancer.

17. Does ovum pickup procedure has complications ?

Basically, any surgical procedure has its risk, but overall the rate of complication during opu is minimal, as it is guided by ultrasound, under anaesthesia.

18. Is the ovum pickup procedure painful ?

No, not generally. It lasts approximately 30 minutes. Some patients have mild cramping or mild abdominal pain after the procedure and are discharged on the same day.

19. Is Embryo transfer a painful procedure ?

Usually embryo transfer is done under ultrasound guidance and it is painless, but in patients with vaginismus we might have to do the embryo transfer under anaesthesia to avoid the discomfort and pain.

20. How many Embryos are transferred ?

In general two embryos are transferred during embryo transfer, but nowadays there is a growing concern for transferring single embryo to restrict the chances of twins.

21. Does the number of embryos influence the chances of pregnancy ?

Earlier it was believed that more number of embryos influences the chances of pregnancy, but now evidence shows that two good quality blastocyst tranfers has the best chance of pregnancy.

22. Can we have sex during treatment ?

Many couples remain intimate during treatment and this is fine, except before a semen sample is asked for ivf/icsi on the day of opu, so it is important to avoid ejaculation for a few days before opu, as this affects both the number of sperm and their motility.

23. Are there risks to having a baby through IVF ?/ Is the incidence of birth defects high ?

Till date, millions of babies have been born around the world, through this technology and the evidence shows there is no statistically significant increase in the incidence of the birth defects.

24. Should I take complete rest once the treatment is started ?

No, complete bed rest is not needed.

25. Does anxiety affects success of IVF ?

Stress and anxiety may cause harmonal imbalance, so throughout the course of IVF better to be calm and relaxed.

26. Is my Uterus healthy enough to carry the baby ?

IVF specialist when they do pelvic ultrasound, they will let you know about your uterus if there is any uterine problems you might have, sometimes surgery may be advised.

27. Are any loans/EMI, available for this treatment for those who are not able pay in single time ?

In India there are few companies which facilitate the the EMI option for IVF treatment, so before you start the treatment it is advisable to talk to your fertility specialist.

28. How much will IVF cost ?

There is no standard fee for IVF treatment as there are a number of factors that will vary for everyone, such as the amount of medication needed. So ask your specialsit for a detailed breakdown of the pricing.

29. Are medications included in the cost of a cycle ?

No, medications are not included in the cost of an IVF cycle. The amount of medication you will need will depend on your age, ovarian reserve and history.

30. Is there any package of treatment ?

Some hospitals do provide a package for IVF treatment. Your IVF cycle package cost would include all monitoring scans, consultation, egg collection, embryo laboratory procedures and an embryo transfer. Drugs and blood tests are charged separately and vary from patient to patient. Some couples may be advised additional tests or procedures like ERA, Hysteroscopy, laparoscopy, TESE/TESA,etc, which will be charged extra.

31. During the process can I travel ?/ Can I work or go to work during IVF ?

Yes, during the process of stimulation of eggs one can travel from home or go to work.

32. Will the first cycle of IVF, be a success for young age women ?

Age is an important factor in IVF, so generally as age progresses the quality of the egg decreases, having IVF in younger age will have the higher success rate.

33. What is the percentage of success with each treatment cycle ?

The possibilities of success with an IVF treatment vary from patient to patient. Your specialist can best predict the outcome in your case after a complete evaluation.

34. what is your clinics success rate on a whole and for patients like me ?

Success rate of individual IVF hospitals very from time to time as success also depends on many factors like patients condition, quality of egg & sperm, and other factors.

35. Can I really become a mother ???/ Is there any chance for me to become pregnant ??

This is one question which is really painful to hear. As doctors we try to do our best, as patient you hav to try the treatment available with trust and hope. So i tell my patients to be positive in approach and be hopefull.

36. What is the IVF Success Rate ?

worldwide success rate of IVF is around 35 to 45%, in the first attempt.

37. Are there any lifestyle changes that might increase our chances of success ?

Yes, Lifestyle changes like quitting smoking and alcohol consumption is advisable. For both husband and wife, a healthy balanced diet rich in fruits & vegetables and exercise helps too. If your BMI is more, it is advisable to reduce the body weight.

38. Will my sugar levels or Thyroid levels affect IVF treatment ?

yes, abnormal sugar levels and abnormal thyroid levels can affect IVF result so it is always advised to keep sugar levels and thyroid levels in normal range before IVF treatment.

39. Does insurance pre approval, takes care of IVF cost ?

Presently in India Insurance is not covering IVF treatment expense.

40. How many chances we can take if IVF becomes a failure ?

Generally most of the infertility patients succeed within first 2 to 3 IVF cycles.

41. What are the options if a woman's own eggs are not producing a pregnancy ?

When a woman's eggs may not be viable and the uterus is healthy and capable of supporting a pregnancy, egg donation with IVF has high success rates.

42. What if I don't respond to the drugs for ovarian stimulation ?

some women do not respond to hormonal injections during egg stimulation, in such patients stimulation will be cancelled and donor egg option will be given.

43. What is the gap period required between 2 IVF cycles after the first unsuccessful IVF ?

It is generally advised to take two to three months of gap after an unsuccessful IVF for the next cycle.

44. Is the incidence, of multifetal pregnancy high ?

Because of 2 embryos transferred in IVF, multiple pregnancy incidence is high.

Egg Donation

45. What is the age criterion for donor selection ?

Preferably 21-29 yrs.

46. How are donors selected ?

A detailed medical, family history is taken along with blood tests for the screening of infectious diseases like HIV, HbsAg, HCV, VDRL.

47. Can we get our own donor ?

No, it has to be from anonymous donor egg program.

48. Are the donors married ?

Donors who are selected will be married and have at least one normal living child.

49. How many eggs are taken from a donor ?

Usually 10-12 eggs.

50. We have been advised to go on the donor sperm, how long will this take and what is the process ?

Most of the IVF hospitals have their own donor bank and can match donors to patients to ensure treatment can be done as quickly as possible. It takes around 1-2 weeks for the process of matching. The embryology team will advise as to how many vials of sperm will be required for your treatment cycle.

51. I have been told I need a Surgical Sperm Retrieval (SSR). What is the chance of obtaining sperm ?

Some men have sperm being produced in their testes, but not present in ejaculate, caused by a blockage, or reduced sperm production. In these cases, we can collect sperm via surgical sperm retrieval. There are 3 methods,

A.TESA- Testicular Sperm Aspiration.

B.TESE- Testicular Sperm Extraction (biopsy).

C.PESA- Percutaneous Epididymal Sperm Aspiration (PESA).

Once sperm has been retrieved, it is used for intracytoplasmic sperm injection (ICSI) to inseminate the collected eggs. But, sometimes we don't manage to retrieve any sper, and in such situation option of donor sperm will be given.

CHAPTER FOUR

DURING IVF

A.Stimulation of eggs

1. How many eggs should be required for good result ?

On an average 10 to 15 eggs will be required ideal for a good result in IVF.

2. How much quality semen should be required from men ?

A good quality semen is also required for good result in IVF, so abstinence of at least 2-3 days is advised before the day of ovum pick up.

3. How many injections do i need for IVF ?

On an average 10 to 12 days of of hormonal injections for stimulation of eggs are necessary, and it varies on patient to patient.

4. Can I Climb stairs during this procedure ?

Yes patients can climb stairs with caution.

5. What are the precautions to be taken during the process ?

To avoid lifting heavy weights, bumpy Road Journeys and to avoid constipation.

6. What are my chances of success in IVF ?

Success depends on many factors, so the treating IVF consultant will be able to tell you about the chances of succes in your case.

7. What can be the side effects or complications I should be prepared for ?

Usually it is mild discomfort or mild pain abdomen.

8. Is there anything about my diagnosis that could negatively impact IVF success ?

The treating doctor will let you know about any negative impact from your past history and diagnosis.

9. How many times do I need to visit the hospital for ultrasounds ?

On an average 4-5 times, if the hormonal injections are taken by yourself at home or else you have to visit continiously daily for injections and scans will be done 4-5 times during your visits.

10. What time should I come to hospital on my 2nd day of menstruation ?

Preferably in the morning hours to visit the hospital.

11. Can I ride 2 wheeler during treatment ?

Yes you can ride the two wheeler or Drive four wheeler but to avoid long and bumpy Road Journeys.

12. Can i inject hormonal injections myself ?

Most injections can be self-administered at your own home, as they are taken subcutaneously. Fertility nurse will show you how to administer the injection so that you are confident with self-injecting, so that you can avoid of your daily hospital visits.

13. Are there any side effects during stimulation ?

Ovarian hyperstimulation syndrome or OHSS can occur when the ovaries are over stimulated with hormonal medicines used in IVF. OHSS symptoms are minor, with mild to moderate pain, loss of appetite, nausea, diarrhoea and feeling bloated.

14. Can I exercise during stimulation period ?

Some mild exercise is acceptable during in-vitro fertilization treatment, but as the IVF treatment cycle progresses the ovaries may become enlarged, and heavy exercise may put you at risk for ovarian torsion, a condition in which the ovary can twist on itself, which is a rare but serious side effect. So, better to avoid gym or heavy exercises.

B.Ovum pick up (opu).

1. How many eggs will you try to retrieve ?

Ideally during the stimulation of eggs when we do a scan we usually tell the patient the number of eggs which are growing depending on the response with hormonal injections for each patient, but it does not mean that whatever number of eggs we see on the ultrasound, all the eggs will be retrieved or aspirated.

We would like to retrieve the maximum possible, but sometimes we end up retrieving no eggs also in conditions called as Empty follicular syndrome. So patient should be well aware of this fact that the number of eggs seen on scanning is not a guarantee that all the eggs will be retrieved, also there is a difference in the growth of each egg, some eggs might not have reached the mature Stage, So we will have to rely only on mature eggs for for the success.

2. Is the egg retrieval procedure painful ?

Because anesthesia is used for egg retrieval, patients feel nothing during the procedure. Egg retrieval is a minor surgery, in which a vaginal ultrasound probe fitted with a long, thin needle is passed through the wall of the vagina into each ovary. The needle punctures each egg follicle and gently removes the egg through a gentle suction. Patients may feel some minor cramping in the ovaries that can be treated with pain medications and will be discharged the same day.

3. Where and how do i produce semen sample ?

Semen samples are delivered by masturbation and can be produced at the hospital in a semen collection room. Men who have had difficulty in producing a semen sample would be advised to produce a semen sample at home and transport it to us within an hour to maintain viability.

4. What happens if my sample is poorer quality than it had been previously ?

We may need to use a procedure called ICSI, where we inject a single sperm into each egg to maximise fertilisation rates, and can be done with very small numbers of sperm. If numbers are extremely low or nil sperm on the day of OPU, we may be able to do a surgical sperm retrieval procedure to recover sperm for treatment.

5. What if I can't produce a sperm sample on the day of treatment ?

Freezing a sample prior to treatment which can be used as a back-up, can help to alleviate stress on the OPU day. If we do not have a semen sample on the day of OPU, we may be able to extract sperm surgically, or Freeze the eggs for later use.

6. When does the treatment start and how long does it take ?

The Ovum pickup procedure is a minor procedure done under anaesthesia, usually it is fixed based on the time of Trigger injection given the day before the procedure. Usually it will be for about 30 minutes and after the procedure patients will be discharge on Day Care basis by the end of the day if no complications.

7. How much rest is required after the procedure ?

Complete bed rest is not necessary after ovum pick up procedure but we do advised to take at least 3 to 4 days of rest at home after the procedure.

8. Can I carry on my normal activities after the procedure ?

Yes all the household normal activities can be carried out after the ovum pick up procedure.

9. Do I need to take leave from work after the procedure?

Leave from work for about 3 to 4 days is advisable after the procedure.

C. IVF/ICSI for fertilisation.

1. How do i know whether my eggs have fertilized ?

Usually after 3 days after your egg collection, embryologist will let you know how many of your eggs have successfully fertilized. Also they will be suggesting about the blastocyst chances for your embryos.

2. Is ICSI better than IVF ?

Yes, ICSI is better than IVF in case of male factor infertility.

D. Blastocyst culture.

1. Is there a chance that none of my embryos will form blastocysts?

Yes, it is possible. Approximately 40-50% of embryos will reach the blastocyst stage and have a higher chance of pregnancy once transferred. In some cases, all of patients' embryos may stop developing at the embryo stage, and results in the embryo transfer been cancelled.

E. Freezing of embryos.

1. For how long we can freeze the embryos ?

Upto 10 yrs, but usually hospitals have yearly or 6 monthly freezing plans.

2. Will the result be affected by longer duration freezing of embryos ?

No, results are not affected by the duration of freezing.

3. In which embryo stage freezing carried out?

Freezing of the embryo can be done at Day 3/5, But freezing at the blastocyst stage is recommended.

4. Are the results of frozen cycle as good as the fresh cycle ?

The results are better in frozen cycle than in fresh cycle.

5. What proportion of embryos survive the freezing/ thawing process ?

This can vary depending on the stage of development that the embryos were frozen and an individual patients' embryos susceptibility to the process. Usually 60-70 % embryos survive.

F. Embryo transfer.

1. Do i need a full bladder for the embryo transfer ?

Yes. When we undertake this procedure we use an ultrasound to view your uterus to check embryo placement. A full bladder provides a clearer view and helps in transfer of embryo in the uterus.

2. How long will the embryo transfer procedure take ?

The complete procedure takes upto 15-20 minutes.

3. What is the minimum endometrium lining thickness you expect before Embryo transfer ?

On 14th day of emdometrial preperation before embryo transfer the minimum endometrial thickness expected is 7 mm.

4. Can I choose for twins/single child during Embryo Transfer ?

Yes before the embryo transfer, you can choose the number of embryos to be transferred. So if you choose one embryo, single embryo will be transfered. But it reduces the success rate and sometimes even with single embryo transfer, there is a chance of having twins also.

5. Will there be anaesthesia before embryo transfer ?

Generally embryo transfer is not done under anaesthesia, but in some patients we do use anaesthesia such as in cases of vaginismus.

6. After the procedure how long she has to be told her urine ?

After the embryo transfer patient will be asked to void the urine after 5 to 10 minutes.

7. How much time do we need to stay in the hospital ?

Patient will be discharged after an hour or two after the ET.

8. Will I be able to freeze my extra embryos ?

Embryos which are not transferred can be frozen if they are of good quality. At the time of embryo transfer the Embryologist will discuss with you the quality of the embryos for transfer and any remaining embryos can be freezed.

9. Is complete bed rest advised after embryo transfer ?

No, complete best rest is not necessary.

10. How much of rest is required immediately post transfer, before one leaves the hospital?

Usually 10-15 mins.

11. What precautions to be after embryo transfer ?

You can do your normal routine household work after transfer, and we would recommend

a. avoiding any heavy lifting.

b. avois strenuous exercise for 2 weeks.

c. avoid straining during defecation.

d. avoid sexual intercourse.

e. avoid climbing stairs frequently.

12. Does one need to take many injections even post transfer ?

This depends on the patient condition.

13. Can I color my hair/nails after embryo transfer ?

It is best to avoid until 12 weeks.

14. What are the diet that I need to follow ?

A healthy balanced diet which is rich in fibre, proteins, fruits and vegetables is advised. Also to avoid foods rich in fat and salt.

15. Does spotting/bleeding occur after ET ?

Some patients may experience spotting pervaginal or mild bleeding after the embryo transfer.

If it is only spotting not to panic.

16. What is the wait time to see the pregnancy positivity after IVF, is it different from normal pregnancy test after missed period ? /How soon after IVF can I do a pregnancy test?

After 14 to 15 days of embryo transfer usually a blood test called as beta HCG is done which says whether you pregnancy is positive.

17. When do I know my confirmation on pregnancy ?

2 weeks after the beta HCG test, when we see fetal heart beat on ultrasound then it is said that the pregnancy is confirmed.

18. Is urine pregnancy test not sufficient to test the result for IVF patient, instead of beta is HCG ?

Urine Pregnancy tests are usually not reliable after IVF, so we do advise to do a blood test after IVF.

19. What is the blood level of beta HCG for it to be positive ?

The values above 100 miu/ml is a good indication that it is a healthy pregnancy.

20. what is beta HCG result to know if the pregnancy is twins ?

Based on the beta HCG value, we may it as having twins or multiple pregnancy if the beta HCG value values are more than 1000 miu/ml, but it is not confirmatory. Only after the ultrasound we can confirm the number of babies.

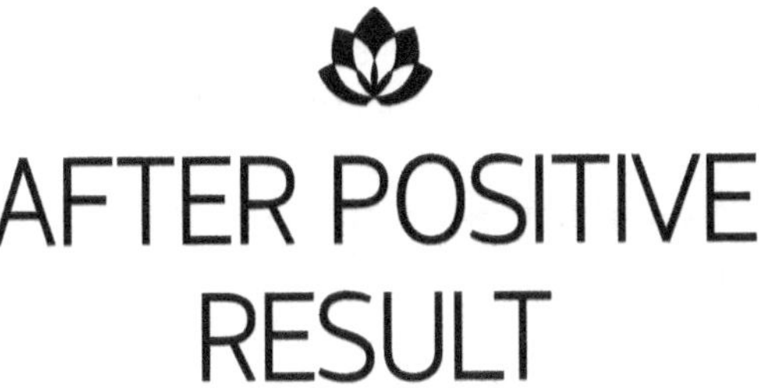

CHAPTER FIVE

AFTER POSITIVE RESULT

1. Does one need to take injections even post positive result ?

It depends on patient to patient.

2. After taking injection there is red spot at the injection spot what to do ?

It is common to have red spot at the injection spot of low molecular weight heparin, so you have to change the site of injection and remain calm.

3. At what frequency pregnancy scans are done ?

We normally carry out your first pregnancy scan two weeks after a positive pregnancy test and then every four weeks after that.

4. When can we have intercourse after I am pregnant ?

If you are pregnant, intercourse is okay after the first confirmatory scan.

5. Is Bus journey better than Train Journey in pregnancy ?

Yes, journey can be done but train Journeys safer than bus.

6. Should i take complete bed rest in pregnancy ?

Not necessary to be on complete bed rest.

7. Does bleeding occurs after pregnancy ?

Some patients may experience bleeding in the early pregnancy but not all spotting or bleeding is bad or going for abortion. Inform your doctor about this symptom and follow the advise.

8. If confirmed with triplets what is the next procedure ?

Triplets may be the result of IVF pregnancy. In case of triplets, patients are advised to go for fetal reduction procedure, where one foetus is reduced by given injection at about 12 weeks so that the other two foetuses grow well till the the delivery.

9. Is my pregnancy going to be normal or c-section ?

Depends on the risk factors patient has after she is pregnant. It is not necessary to have C section for all IVF patients but it depends on other factors.

10. Does the ivf doctor will be along till delivery or should we have to check for other doctor for delivery ?

It depends on the hospital you are taking treatment. Most of the IVF hospitals do have facilities for the delivery but if the delivery facility is not available then the IVF doctor may refer you to other obstetrician after two to three months.

11. IVF pregnancy is a risk always. is it a myth or true ?/Is IVF pregnancy different with regard to delivery, scans any other test taken by normally conceived women ?

Yes IVF pregnancy is same as Natural pregnancy.

12. Can I start with pregnancy Yoga ?

Yes one can practice mild yoga or mild exercises during pregnancy.

13. Is there a higher risk of miscarriage in IVF treatment ?

Miscarriage risk of IVF pregnant patients are similar to normally conceived pregnant patients.

14. Is any particular diet recommended ?

A healthy balanced diet rich in proteins, fibres, fruits and vegetables are advised.

15. What should be the sleeping posture ?

Left lateral position is better for sleeping.

16. what is a safe and healthy pregnancy delivery week for twin IVF pregnancy ?

34 completed gestational weeks are safe for twin IVF pregnancies.

17. Will the amount of medicines or injections hormone effect post delivery ?

No, the amount of medications or injections used during IVF will not be a problem post delivery.

18. Will spotting or mild bleeding after 15 days post pregnancy test means miscarriage even after taking all medicines/injections ?

No just spotting after embryo transfer does not mean it is miscarriage.

CHAPTER SIX

AFTER RESULT IS NEGATIVE

1. What s the beta HCG value, which indicates it is negative ?

Beta HCG value of less than 5 miu/ml indicates that it is negative result.

2. My beta HCG value is 35 miu/ml, what to do ?

In some patients the value of beta HCG is less than 100 miiu/ml but greater than 5 miu/ml, in such cases, we do recommend to repeat the blood test every 48 hours. If repeated test value doubles in value every 48 hours then the pregnancy may be healthy. If the values fall after 48 hours then it is said that it is Biochemical pregnancy.

3. What are causes of my failure ?

Cause of IVF failure, may be related to embryo quality or egg/sperm quality, uterine factor or genetic,etc.

4. Why not baby growing even after blood positive ?

May be the implantation took place, but the growth of foetus is affected by one of the many factors of failure.

5. How soon can you do IVF after failed cycle ?

We advise that you allow your body to rest for 2-3 months before commencing another cycle.

Thank you again for reading this book. I hope this book was able to help you to find the answers for most of your questions. The next step is to get your doctor and discuss your options and start the treatment.

If you enjoyed this book please take the time to share your thoughts and post a review on Amazon, it would be greatly appreciated.

If any queries, do write a mail to **vinodlongi@gmail.com**

Thank you and i wish you both ALL THE BEST.

BE POSITIVE AND BE HOPEFUL.